Hi, my name is Darryl. I want to share with you one of the most interesting, versatile, unknown and widely needed resources EVERYONE should have in their home arsenal. Please read EVERTHING and consult a physician before trying anything recommended in this book. Oh yeah, even though these remedies work, none of them have been approved by the USFDA. After reading this I know you're going to be so anxious to get started, so please, please take it slowly, follow the advice of your doctor, do your own research, follow the recipes closely, and PAY ATTENTION to what you're doing and how your body responds…!!

Let's get started. I've been interested in herbal medicine and natural remedies since I was in elementary school. I've always been into using what's around me to my advantage. Taking things in nature and giving it a purpose. Ever since I heard my uncle mention this one particular root, my imagination and curiosity has been set ablaze. That root, was Ginseng. When I heard how many benefits this plant had and all the wonderful things it could do, I INSTANTLY fell in love.

Ginseng is an adaptogen. That means it helps the body adapt to stressful moments in life and helps the body balance itself. This herb can help your body to reset itself and be more productive. And this is not the only herb that does this. There are many other herbs that help the body to reduce stress and fight toxins to keep the body in balance naturally and without side effects.

From then on, the mention of ginseng sends me into a flurry. It causes my passion for homeopathic cures to set itself on fire. My passion for creating different herbal remedies that actually work starts to kick my brain into overdrive. I REALLY enjoy finding different ways to use the simple, healthy, inexpensive herbs God placed on this planet for us to use. This is one way to stay healthy and save money at the same time.

You can drink a simple cup of herbal tea, more commonly known as tisane, or create an herbal seasoning, or even make your own herbal sauces and marinades for the foods you eat. If you're serious about being healthy and keeping natural herbs as a part of your life, keep reading to learn a whole new world of staying healthy and creating natural cures.

At the time I am writing this, I am a 33 year old male with 3 bachelor degrees in communications, with a masters and PhD level training in counseling. I have been living with a spinal disability since 2006. I have spinal stenosis. Spinal stenosis is an abnormal narrowing of the spinal canal that may occur in any of the regions of the spine.

This narrowing causes a restriction to the spinal canal, resulting in a neurological deficit. Symptoms include pain, numbness, and loss of motor control. For me, the daily pain from this deficit, not being able to afford doctors or medication, and my love for natural remedies is what drove me to find an herbal solution to my problem.

I have helped numerous people make money; find their way in life; start and build healthy families and business; mentored and educated children and adults; and help many MANY people change their diets, eating habits, and overall health which in turn changed their thinking process, motivation, prosperity and overall way of life. The key to making ANY kind of change in life is to know and admit a change needs to be made. After knowing and admitting, that's where THIS information comes in handy.

I'm not saying that herbal tea, tisane, is the know-all – heal-all of the world. What I'm saying is that by admitting you have things in your life that need to be changed you can use herbal teas as a STARTING point to changing ANYTHING that's troubling you in your life.

The reason being, is that each herb has specific properties and functions. Some herbs help you relax, think better, increase blood flow, give you energy and much MUCH more. Knowing these functions and properties in turn helps you to create a map that will allow you to figure out exactly what's ailing you and to determine exactly how to fix it. Once you admit something needs to be changed, you can start working on that roadmap to healthy living and thinking — which will change your life FOREVER.

Best of all — what I'm proposing to you is not something you fix and it comes back over and over again... What

I'm suggesting is to create and use a system that will allow you to continuously resolve issues in your life as they come up and, regardless of whether they are new or old issues, this system will continue to produce positive results as long as you use it. This system will let you customize everything to your particular problem, need and health situation. Plus, this system is EASY to use anytime and anywhere – mix ahead of time and carry it with you.

First, figure out the problem you're having in your life. You can't fix something if it isn't broken. Second, admit that it's a problem that needs to be changed – the first step in overcoming ANY situation is admitting that it exists. I have known people with

PROVEN medical issues who DO NOT believe there is a problem no matter how much evidence their doctor gives. Third, allow yourself to come up with solutions – meaning come up with ways to SOLVE THE PROBLEM. A lot of the time people address and fix the symptoms and not the problem – symptoms are temporary; problems are permanent; if left unhandled. Fourth, research herbs and their functions. The more you are familiar with herbs and what they do for your body, the better you will become at being able to resolve issues; not only in your life, but in the lives of those around you. Lastly, stock up on the herbs you use the most. By having a stockpile of herbs for general and personal use, when you combine it with your continued research you can come up with a healthy solution to ANY problem ANYTIME you need one. So, just by making a simple cup of tea, you can do anything you set your mind to.

Now-a-days, when people think about tea, they think about some fast food place that gives it to you for $1 a cup or a $5 box with 10 bags that people drop into hot cups of water. These teas are usually made from green, black or white tea leaves and are mainly grown and picked for a particular flavor. The 'tea' that we are talking about when we are talking about *'herbal tea'* is something completely different. It's not 'tea' at all; 'tea' is the term used for the particular brewing process used to make herbal tea.

Tisane, or "herbal tea", is a term for any non-caffein beverage made from the infusion or decoction of herbs, spices, or other plant material. These drinks are distinguished from caffeinated beverages like coffee, maté and the true teas (black, green, white, yellow, oolong, etc.). In addition to serving as a beverage, many tisanes are also consumed due to a perceived medicinal benefit. Like brews made from the tea bush, such infusions are prepared by combining hot water and fruits, leaves, roots or grains. The resulting drink can be served hot or cold.

Brewing *herbal* tea, or tisane, is the same as brewing a regular cup of tea, the only difference is the length of time needed to make a perfect cup. Regular tea takes anywhere from 2-5 minutes to steep the tea leaves. Depending on the type of herb and whether its fresh, dried or powdered, brewing a tisane could take anywhere from 10-30 minutes to get all the medicinal values from the ingredients.

There are more ways to extract the medicine from the herbs; tinctures, presses or raw consumption; but the easiest and most well know way is to drink it in teat format – cup + herb + boiling water = tea. This format of tea making has been around since the beginning of tea making. Tisanes have been used for nearly as long as written history extends. Documents have been recovered dating back to as early as Ancient Egypt and Ancient China that discuss the enjoyment and uses of tisanes. It is the best way to get the maximum results you need from your herbs without having to get an industrial press or brewing equipment.

Finding the herbs you like and brewing them yourself is the best thing you can do for your family, yourself and for your budget. It's also fun and educational too. There are so many things you can learn about these herbs and yourself from doing the research. You can learn how to heal ANYTHING that ails you just by researching and keeping herbs available.

******NOTE ABOUT HERBS******

CONSULT A PHYSICIAN

BEFOR STARTING ANY HERBAL REGIMEN

It will be helpful to know that if you use whole herbs, whether dried or fresh, that there is a difference when using the root and the flower/leaves. Roots are thicker so it will take longer to steep(20-30 minutes) than the flowers/leaves(10-15 minutes). Depending on the herb, sometimes roots are better, flowers are better, or leaves are better. PLEASE DO THE RESEARCH! Knowledge is POWER so equip yourself to be as powerful as possible.

There is also a significant difference between using dried and fresh herbs for your tea. Some herbs have different qualities based on whether or not they are used fresh, dried whole or dried and powdered. While you do your research, make sure you pay attention to how much benefit you get in each state. Sometimes it will be easy, and better, to get fresh herbs and sometimes just more convenient to do powdered. Plus, the herbs will last for different periods of time in each form – that's VERY important.

For ALL recipes in this manual, the herbs will be dried and powdered.

After finding the herbs that are right for you, you have to know how to handle them properly to make the most out of your herbal supply. Though there are more methods to doing this, we're only going to talk about making tea. As stated earlier, making tea is really easy. The equation for tea is: cup + herb + water = tea. To make the perfect cup, you need a few things:

measuring spoons - ½ teaspoon (tsp); 1 teaspoon (tsp); 1 tablespoon (tbsp)

8 oz tea cup or coffee mug

wire strainer

2-quart (qt) sauce pan

sweetener – sugar; honey; lemon; whatever you like

herbs (1ST MOST IMPORTANT)

water (2ND MOST IMPORTANT)

*****A NOTE ABOUT SWEETNER*****

When choosing a sweetener PLEASE remember that you don't need to overdo it. The point of drinking the tea is to get the health benefits. Adding too much sweetener is DEFINITELY a killer of the healthy aspect of the tea. PLEASE remember to use them with care.

There are herbs you can buy to use as a sweetener, like mint, spearmint, or stevia and many others; try using one of those. Using herbs to sweeten herbal tea is a good way to get even more benefits because the herbal sweeteners have medicinal benefits too. Sometimes you will need to add sugar. Use more than one sweetener so that you cut down the amount of sugar.

The best sweetener combination I personally have found is stevia and sugar. Stevia is 30-300 times sweeter than sugar. But by itself, stevia is totally earthy tasting. So you need to use something else to bring out that sweetness (if not sugar, use honey). I pre-make the stevia/sugar mix and use a ration of 1tbsp of stevia to 1tsp sugar or 1 full part of stevia to 1/3 part of sugar. Mix evenly. Add to taste.

After you have assembled your supplies and ingredients, take you tea cup or coffee mug, fill it with water, and pour it into your sauce pan twice. Bring to a boil. While the water is boiling, measure 1/2 tsp of each herb into your cup (no more than 4 –or– 2tsp of matter per 8 ounces). When the water starts boiling, take the pot off the heat, count to 10 slowly, then pour the herbs from your cup directly into the water. Let the herbs steep for 10-15 minutes for leaves/flowers, or 20-30 minutes for roots/grains, while stirring every 2-3 minutes (stirring releases the medicinal properties and cools the tea at the same time).

Once the tea has set for long enough, you can either strain it with the wire strainer and sweeten or you can just go straight to sweetening it without straining. Straining and not straining do have their own individual benefits. RESEARCH!!!!!!!

Now we talk about safety. When dealing with heat and herbs, it is always best to use the utmost caution possible. Primarily one would think the heat is the most important safety hazard, but the herbs come first – but still use as much caution as possible when using ANY source of heat. The main reason the herbs are most important is because without the herbs, you have nothing but a hot cup of water and no reason for doing anything else.

The main concerns for your herbs are freshness, potency and foreign objects. Even if you're using dried or powdered material it's very important to know how fresh your herbs really are. Out of date herbs can lose their potency; potency in flavor and medicinal efficacy, rendering them useless. Using non-fresh or spoiled herbs can be just as bad as using the wrong herb or over doing it.

With some herbs, you need to know how strong the medicines in them are. Many herbs are very beneficial as medicine, but the medicinal aspects should be measured based on extraction, effect on the body, and how they're consumed. Herbs perform better and have different strengths using different extraction processes. As for our method, tea or tisane, water dilutes and sometimes does not get all of the medical properties out.

To some this is not good, but for us, this makes it ideal for slow daily intake, which in turn makes it perfect for preventive measures, daily health management, and long-term treatment. Plus, water is the world's BEST natural cleanser for the body. Just remember that with most herbs, even though it's not as strong as it could be, some effects are still strong enough and immediate.

For daily consumers, it is recommended, though, that for every 8 weeks of daily use you DO NOT consume any herbs for 1 full week. The reason for this is because your body will adapt to herbs after a certain period of time. This lowers your tolerance to the medicinal value, which causes the herbs to be ineffective. This week of non-use gives your body a chance to flush out the herbs and reset so that you can continue to get the full benefit from them.

Last, but DEFINITELY a very important factor, is the risk of foreign objects. We need to talk beyond the obvious dirt and rocks and what not. Those are important, but when it comes to herbs, what you can't see is more important than what you can see.

The good thing is that you will never have to worry about those things if you purchase from quality vendors you can trust, store your herbs properly, and make sure your water gets to a boil before you pour it over your herbs. The best way to store herbs is by placing them in a moisture-free air-tight container at room temperature (definitely not over the stove, in the refrigerator, or next to an air vent).

Next let's talk about a couple of herbs that you can start to use immediately to kick-off this new system we're creating. These herbs will be used to help you gain more energy and bring internal balance. Once these herbs start to take effect you will notice the difference – almost immediately.

You will have more energy. You will think clearer. You will have more endurance. Your brain functions will increase. Your body's internal workings will flush and cleanse itself allowing you to accept thoughts clearly and use this new found energy more efficiently. You will start to feel better. It will not happen overnight(well...it might...teeheehee!), but it will happen and you will feel it.

The herbs we will be working with are ginseng (2 types), epimedium, muira puama, spearmint and stevia. When we are finished, this concoction will be a sweet, minty, energy bomb that you can pull out anytime you need an extra kick. This particular combination will give you lots of energy, cleanse you, help you think better, and bring you back into balance physically and mentally. Now we have to learn about each herb.

We're going to start with my personal favorite – ginseng. As stated before, ginseng is an adaptogen, which means it brings your body into balance and helps you adapt to stress. It gets it's stress fighting properties from elements called ginsenosides. Ginseng has been regarded as a heal-all type of herb because the yin and yang qualities possessed by those classified as ginsengs. Its ability to bring the body and mind into focus has been studied and researched for many decades.

There are a few different types of ginseng. Each type has its own specific benefits even though most of them work exactly the same. The only way to know if it's true ginseng is to look at its scientific categorization. True ginseng is of the genus Panax. Many of the plants classified as ginseng are really not 'ginseng' at all, but because they have the same characteristics as ginsenosides and have general adaptogenic effects, they are classified as ginsengs.

One particular plant that mimics traditional ginseng, almost perfectly, is called Siberian Ginseng. The scientific name, *Eleutherococcus senticosus*, puts this plant into another classifying group. But research shows that 'Siberian ginseng' has almost the exact same benefits as standard ginseng, or Panax Ginseng. Siberian ginsengs have eleutherosides, which work just like ginsenosides. Even though they are different chemically, the effects are the same. They both provide extra endurance, cleansing of the mind and body, provide anti-oxidants, relieve pain and much much more. That's why these herbs are considered to be 'heal-all' types of herbs.

These next 2 herbs may not be as versatile as ginseng, but their beneficial effects are sometimes stronger. These herbs are mainly used to increase blood flow and relieve pain. Increasing blood flow allows the body to use oxygen more efficiently. Brain functions increase, muscle endurance increases, and stamina dramatically increases with these 2 plants – epimedium (horny goat weed) and muira puama (potency wood).

Epimedium, best known as 'horny got weed' is highly know for it aphrodisiac effects. But, it is because of these aphrodisiac properties that make it a medicinal benefit. When taken, epimedium increases blood flow by allowing certain muscles to relax and blood vessels to open so that the blood flows through the body much easier.

Muira puama does the same thing. Muira puama, also known as 'potency wood' is another aphrodisiac type herb that has wonderful medicinal benefits vastly similar to epimedium, horny goat weed. The nickname, potency wood, should say it all. This herbs has much stronger effects than epimedium.

Think of it like this, epimedium is the starter class and muira puama is the finishing class. When combined together, these 2 herbs can do wonders for the human body. This combination increases energy levels, stamina, oxygen flow, allowing for better pain relief, a cleaner system, and the ability to do more for longer.

The ability to do more comes from the increase in the delivery of blood through the body. This helps to maintain better healthy oxygen levels to the heart, brain and nervous system, provide muscle longevity, and increase mental and physical stamina, and the ability to relieve aches and pains caused by the stresses of life. This gives you the natural energy to do more, longer and more efficiently without hurting the body or causing any negative side effects – and that's what we want right; a body that does more, lives longer and works at its top performance without pain.

It seems that in nature, most of the time, the healthier something is for us, the more it tastes like crap. In all honesty, to be able to drink these herbal teas straight with no sweetener is an acquired taste – a taste that not all people can actually acquire. And, it seems that if it doesn't taste good, people are not going to eat or drink it. That's why our next subject to talk about is about sweetener.

Sweeteners are substances that appeal to the sweet part of our taste buds. In order for something bad to taste good, sometimes the best thing to do is make it taste sweeter. Most of the time when people want to make something sweeter they automatically reach for the sugar. I'm not saying that sugar itself is bad; because it's not. Sugar is just misunderstood. Our bodies need sugar so we MUST consume it. But it's the types of sugars, what foods we get them from, and how much we eat that really makes the difference. When it comes to herbal tea, the more sugar you use, the less benefit it has. Because the sugar changes the chemical properties and weakens the medicinal properties, its best to use a little as possible.

Most of the time, you'll need to add a little bit of sugar to offset the natural flavors of the herbs – but like I said, YOU ONLY NEED A LITTLE. When choosing sweeteners it is important to choose one with the right flavor that won't need much of anything else to make it better. And if you really need to use something else, try to use another herb; something that also has medicinal benefits as well as sweetening properties. That's why I chose these 2 particular herbs as sweeteners – stevia and spearmint.

Stevia is n herb that is anywhere between 30-300 times sweeter than sugar without using any form of sugar. Stevia takes a little longer than sugar to activate the sweet receptors in your mouth, but that sweet flavor lasts longer on your tongue than sugar does. Stevia has been the center of many studies as a sweetener for people with diabetes, or people on carbohydrate-controlled diets, because it doesn't contain the glucose present in sugar, therefore, controlling blood-sugar levels better. Even the popular cola companies have started to use the sweetening powers of stevia – maybe you should too…!

The next great herb to talk about for sweetening teas is one that is pretty popular for taste but unknown for medicine. Many folks didn't even realize that this herb, spearmint, had any medicinal properties at all. Most people know spearmint for its flavor in candies and gum, but spearmint has been used for centuries for making things taste good and keeping people healthy.

Spearmint is in the mint family. It is considered to be weaker in minty flavor than most other mints like its big brother, peppermint. As well as having a great flavor, spearmint has been used for its carminative properties. What that means is that it helps your stomach to prevent making gas or helps it to get rid of gas. In other words spearmint has been used through history as a digestive aid. Spearmint also has anti-fungal, antioxidant and calming properties. Its soothing effect works well for insomnia and massages. From an herbal point of view, spearmint isn't just for gum and candy canes anymore...

The best thing you can do for yourself when it comes to herbal sweeteners is trial and error. The reason I put it like that is because some herbs have a stronger flavor than others. You really want to actively pay close attention to the amount of sweetener you use with certain herbs, whether used individually or mixed. Even though the sweet herbs I mentioned have healthy benefits, using too much can be just as bad as using sugar.

Please, please, take the time to do the research into what you like and what it takes to get the most benefit out of the herbs you use. A lot of the reason that people do not eat healthy or live healthy lifestyles is because they don't pay attention to the internal things that

that make us happy and help us to grow. Our minds and bodies should be the most important pieces of equipment we have so it should be especially important to keep this equipment in tip-top condition for best performance.

Paying attention to our bodies is the most important key to living healthy lives. The better we keep track of our bodies the better they work; the more you can do; the better you feel; the more you enjoy life – and that's the most important thing, RIGHT!

And that's it!! You are now a professional home herbal tea brewer. If you follow the system I just outlined, you'll have everything you need to solve any problem in your life. There is nothing like a simple cup of tea to help you relax, unwind, let the blood flow and allow your thoughts to run wild, or not to run at all.

Herbal tea can fix almost ANYTHING that's wrong by either helping you get to the solution, or by actually providing the solution to the problem medicinally. So remember, cup + herb + water = tea and research, Research, RESEARCH!! Thank you for joining me on this herbal journey; stay well, stay blessed and MUCH LOVE!!

References

www.google.com

www.mountainroseherbs.com

www.wikipedia.org

www.raysahelian.com

www.webmd.com

www.ask.com